I0487378

My Bilateral Knee Replacement

My Bilateral Knee Replacement

A Personal Story

By Ann Nohava
as told by her daughters Patty Melton,
Barb Martin and Susan Culp

Writers Club Press
San Jose New York Lincoln Shanghai

My Bilateral Knee Replacement
A Personal Story

All Rights Reserved © 2001 by Ann Nohava

No part of this book may be reproduced or transmitted in any
form or by any means, graphic, electronic, or mechanical,
including photocopying, recording, taping, or by any
information storage retrieval system, without the permission in
writing from the publisher.

Writers Club Press
an imprint of iUniverse.com, Inc.

For information address:
iUniverse.com, Inc.
5220 S 16th, Ste. 200
Lincoln, NE 68512
www.iuniverse.com

Credits to Patty Melton, Barb Martin, Susan Culp
No portion of this book may be used without the author's prior
permission.

ISBN: 0-595-19219-X

Printed in the United States of America

Contents

Preface

This is my personal story of my bilateral total knee replacement. I, along with my three daughters, wrote this book for two reasons. The first reason is to inform people about what they can expect from bilateral knee replacement surgery as opposed to surgery on one knee at a time. But more importantly, the second reason for this book is to provide as much information as possible to anyone contemplating this type of surgery before they go forward with it.

The anxieties you have before major surgery are so different than the ones you have after surgery. Often, people think that once the surgery is over, the worries and pain are over. Instead, it can be the beginning of a different set of worries and pain. But, if you know in advance what to expect, you can plan accordingly and will have a much easier time after your operation.

There are many books out there with regard to one total knee replacement, but very little about a bilateral—meaning two—knee replacement. We want to tell you all the facts that could occur, and in my case, did occur, before a very large decision such as this one is made.

You should try to read up on this type of surgery and get all the information you can about your surgeon, the hospital, the anesthesiologist, the care center, the potential problems that can arise, the tremendous pain before surgery from arthritis, the excruciating pain after surgery, the depression that ensued in my case, and after approximately nine months, the happiness I felt that I had opted for bilateral surgery rather than one knee surgery at a time.

I would like to add that not everyone should do as is written in this book regarding my particular case. Everyone is different and has different needs. This is merely an account of my condition and subsequent surgery and I am writing this only to inform and educate you. I was not prepared emotionally or physically for what would happen to me. I am recommending that anyone considering a knee replacement research as much as possible in advance of his or her surgery. I hope that in writing this, I save one person from some of the unknown that I experienced.

List of Contributors

Patty Melton, Barb Martin, Susan Culp

Introduction

I was very lucky and most everything came out ok, but I should not have had such severe surgery without some research.

I did not explore anything before I had my knee replacement surgery. My knees had been painful for me for years and were progressing rapidly to the surgery stage. I had taken so many over-the-counter pain pills over the years, but nothing was easing the pain. As the pain got worse I had x-rays taken and my internist suggested I go see an orthopedic surgeon for further consultation. My first impression of this surgeon was positive—his demeanor, humor, and most importantly his knowledge. I was completely satisfied with him. I had not gone to him with the instant thought of total knee replacement. As a matter of fact, my only concern was to stop the pain. I was wondering if he could give me a cortisone shot to ease the pain. I had one shot in the right knee and it immediately eased the pain.

He looked at the x-rays that had been taken at the internists telling me that my knees were in pretty bad shape—bone touching bone already. At that time, my right knee hurt much more than the left and before I left the office I felt great. I thought that this surely was the way to go. Approximately three months later the pain reoccurred. So I returned to the surgeon for another shot. After six months I needed another shot, but this time I received shots in both legs and again, nine months later, I received once again shots in both legs. Needless to say, the pain was getting worse. The cortisone was hiding the pain temporarily, but the problem was still there. A year after my first cortisone shot, it seemed as if the pain overcame the shots way too fast and the shots weren't helping anymore. We began talking about surgery.

I decided at this time that surgery was my only option. As mentioned earlier, I ignorantly did no research. My oldest daughter did as much research as possible, but she could not find anything to read on a bilateral knee replacement. I have an older brother who had had surgery—one leg at a time— and when I indicated that I would prefer to do both and get it over with, his comment to me was that I should not do that and that I wouldn't be able to stand all the pain that goes along with this particular surgery. "Please Ann, only do one leg at a time."

My idea was do them both and get it over with. I reasoned with myself that I would only have one recuperation period, would only need to be off work once, not twice, and would only have one set of expenses, not two. My internist also was not too thrilled that I wanted bilateral surgery, because of all the things I have previously mentioned. Because of his comments, I then decided one leg at a time. So we scheduled surgery.

The day before surgery the surgeon looked at the new x-rays showing me the terrible shape both of my old knees were in, but I now had bone spurs to add to the problem. The surgeon's comment to me was, "If I can get the scheduled time I would need at the hospital, should we go forward with a bilateral knee replacement?" I was taken aback. This is what I had wanted in the first place, then had changed my mind after a time, and now here we were at the crossroads. Finally, in the long run, my surgeon helped me decide definitely on having both legs operated on. While we were talking about recuperation time, he mentioned that often times people do not come back for the second operation after having the first operation and experiencing all the pain that goes along with the healing procedure of the operation. They just did not want to go through that pain again. So I decided that I wanted to proceed. When he found he could have the time and space at the hospital, it was set. I look back and think, maybe a person should be really concerned or nervous, but all I could think of at the time was to get it over with, so I could walk again. The pain I would experience after surgery, if the surgery would be successful, or any complications from the surgery, never entered my mind. I knew it would be just fine! I hope you find this book interesting and very helpful in making your decision.

Chapter One

The Pain

A painful knee can gravely affect your ability to lead a full active life, as it did mine. Over the last several years, major advancements in artificial knee replacements have greatly improved the outcome of surgery and as a result, artificial knee replacement surgery is becoming more and more common as the population of the world begins to age.

Joint replacements have made significant contributions to millions of people by providing relief of pain, improved function and increased enjoyment of life. It must be remembered though, that successful as the surgery may be, the knee replacement is not a normal joint and requires special care and consideration. The success of your total knee replacement depends on your determination to achieve the best results possible, both through immediate after surgery care and rehabilitation and your long-term care. The success of your joint replacement depends on you. Each person is unique and the surgeon and therapist may make specific recommendations for individual cases.

There are many causes and conditions that result in degeneration of the knee joint. Osteoarthritis is the most common cause for patients who have knee replacement surgery. Osteoarthritis is commonly referred to as wear and tear arthritis. Osteoarthritis can occur with no previous injury to the knee joint—the knee simply wears out. Some people may have a genetic tendency that increases their chances of developing osteoarthritis.

The major problem in osteoarthritis is that the cartilage on the surface of the bone inside the joint wears away. Once the slick protective surface of this cartilage is worn away, the result is bone rubbing against bone, which is very painful.

Fractures of the knee, torn cartilage, and torn ligaments can also cause the knee joint to function abnormally. This abnormal function can lead to excessive wear and tear of the joint many years after the injury.

I had the most common symptom of a degenerative knee joint, which was pain. You will notice this symptom begin usually while bearing weight on the affected knee, such as when walking. You may start to limp, gradually at first, and finally with almost every move until it is difficult to make it through a shopping excursion or up a flight of stairs without shortness of breath. Your knee may become swollen with fluid. Your range of motion of the affected knee can be affected and the knee will slowly and eventually bend less than normal and may lose its ability to completely straighten out. Bone spurs will usually develop and can be seen on an x-ray. Finally, as your condition worsens, you may feel pain almost all of the time, day and night.

At this point most patients who have been putting up with the pain will now see a doctor, because the pain is fast becoming unbearable. The diagnosis of a degenerative knee joint starts with a complete history and physical examination by your surgeon. X-rays are required to determine how bad your knee joint has become. X-rays may help suggest a cause for the degeneration in your knee. Other tests may be required if your surgeon thinks that other conditions may be adding to the degenerative process. Blood tests can rule out systemic arthritis, such as rheumatoid arthritis, or an infection in the knee.

Not all degenerative knee conditions require a knee replacement as a first treatment. Your doctor may suggest several alternative treatments to put off replacing the knee as long as possible. Anti-inflammatory medicines may reduce the inflammation from the arthritis and reduce pain. Cortisone shots, such as mine, will also relieve much of the pain.

But, most degenerative problems will eventually require replacement of the painful knee with an artificial knee joint, called a prosthesis. The decision to proceed with surgery should be made by you, your family, and your doctor and only after you feel that you understand as much as possible about the surgery and recovery process.

Chapter Two

The Knee

The knee joint is a complex, hinge-type joint that relies on strong ligaments and muscles for stability and support. Movement occurs in flexion and extension (bending and straightening) only. The ligaments on either side of the joint prevent unwanted sideways movements. There are three surfaces in the knee joint: the lower end of the thighbone, the upper end of the shinbone, and a kneecap.

The ends of two or more bones that are connected by thick tissues form a joint. For example, the lower leg bone (tibia or shin bone) and the thighbone (femur) form the knee joint. The bone ends of a joint are covered with a smooth layer called cartilage. Healthy cartilage allows nearly frictionless and pain-free movement, but when damaged or diseased by arthritis, joints become stiff and painful. A fibrous tissue envelope encloses every joint with a smooth tissue lining called the synovium, which produces fluid that reduces friction and wear to the joint.

Joint replacement surgery is considered only for those people with severely damaged joints that can no longer be successfully managed by other means (e.g.: medications or exercise). Surgery is performed for the following reasons:

- To relieve pain (the primary reason in the majority of people)
- To improve function, e.g. walking, sitting, climbing stairs
- To improve joint movement
- To improve alignment and correct deformity
- To improve stability

The purpose of joint replacement is to relieve the pain in the joint caused by the damage done to the cartilage. Pain may be so severe a person may avoid using the joint, which weakens the muscles around the joint and makes it even more difficult to move the joint.

Total joint replacement will be considered after other treatment options do not relieve pain and disability. Surgery will replace the damaged parts of the joint. For example: for an arthritic knee, damaged ends of the bones and cartilage are replaced with metal and plastic surfaces shaped to restore knee movement and function. For an arthritic hip, the damaged ball is replaced by a metal ball attached to a metal stem fit into the femur, and a plastic socket is implanted into the pelvis, replacing the damaged socket.

Hip and knee replacements are the most common, however, joint replacement can be performed on other joints, including the ankle, foot, shoulder, elbow and fingers.

The artificial knee joint is called a prosthesis. There are two main types of artificial knee replacements: cemented prosthesis and uncemented prosthesis. Both types are widely used. In many cases, a combination of the two types is used. The kneecap, or patellar, portion of the prosthesis is usually cemented into place. The choice to use a cemented or uncemented prosthesis is usually made by the surgeon based on your age and lifestyle, and your surgeon's experience.

Each prosthesis has four parts. The tibial component replaces the end of the tibia. The tibia is commonly called the shinbone. The femoral component replaces the end of the femur, the groove where the kneecap slides. The femur is commonly called the thighbone. It is the largest bone in the body. The patellar component replaces the surface on bottom of the patella. The "top" of the kneecap is the part you can feel through your skin. The "bottom" is the on the other side, and slides up and down in the femoral groove whenever you bend or straighten your leg.

The femoral component is made of metal. The tibial component is usually made of two parts—a metal tray that is fit directly onto the bone and a plastic spacer that provides a bearing surface. The plastic used is very tough and very slick—so slick and tough that you could ice skate on this sheet of the plastic without much damage to the plastic.

A cemented prosthesis is held in place using an epoxy type cement that attaches the metal to the bone. An uncemented prosthesis has a fine mesh of holes on the surface that allows the bone to grow into the mesh and attaches the prosthesis to the bone. The materials used in a total joint replacement are designed to enable the joint to move just like a normal joint. Several metals are used, including stainless steel, alloys of cobalt and chrome, and titanium. The plastic material is durable and wear resistant polyethylene. A plastic bone cement may be used to anchor the prosthesis into the bone. Joint replacements also can be implanted without cement when the prosthesis and the bone are designed to fit and lock together directly.

The majority of people experience good to excellent results following knee replacement. This means significant relief of pain and improved functional movement and strength. This enables them to walk, sit, drive a car and cope with the activities of daily life more easily.

The life of the replacement is difficult to predict but is generally 12 to 15 years. The rate of wear on the plastic is so minimal that "wearing out" is not a factor.

Chapter Three

My background

(As told by my daughters)

For as long as we can really remember my mom had bad knees. She always had a hard time getting off the floor. We remember when we were young that she would play or do puzzles with us and have to work at getting off of the floor. That was probably the start of it as we can remember it. At its worst, she could not get through a grocery store without gasping for air, holding onto a shopping cart and being in excruciating pain. Any kind of errand was a task. She could not go up a flight of three steps to her townhouse without wincing in pain. She could not bend her knees to climb up one leg at a time—she would go one foot up, the other to that step, rest a second, the first foot up the next step, the other one following to the same step, rest a second and so on. Things were slow going. People would tell her she needed to walk and get exercise—which would be the best thing for her. My goodness, she could barely walk to her car from her front door. How was she supposed to take a walk? We were successful in getting her a handicapped sticker for her car, and this helped her tremendously. All of this happened so gradually over a period of 30 years, that her arthritis and pain became a part of how we thought of her. But it was time for us to do something about it. So when she decided to have her knees replaced, we were all for it. Although we prided ourselves on being the type of people who did their homework, read articles, talked to doctors and researched material pertaining to the situation, nothing prepared us or our family for the emotions we would all encounter from this operation.

As we had known, damage could occur in the knee joint for a variety of reasons. It could occur from injury to the bones or by some disease process, which may produce joint damage such as arthritis. Some forms of arthritis may involve only the knee joints. In others, the knee problem may be one part of a more widespread disease process. In my mom's case, arthritis had caused irreparable damage to her knees.

The most serious symptom she experienced was increasing pain, particularly when bearing weight through the joint, but also at rest. Motion was gradually lost, and the remaining movement was rough and the result was the loss of her ability to function normally. Walking was slow going and she plugged along, but when mom finally stopped doing things with her family because she was too tired, or she thought she would slow us down or just did not think she could keep up, we knew it was time for us to consider something that would take her out of her pain. She was only 67, and this was much too young in my mom's case for her to stop the activities that she always had done.

Six months before my mom's knee replacement surgery we read a book on hip and knee replacements. We personally needed to understand as closely as possible what the procedure entailed. It was the only literature on the surgery that we had read, and wished there had been more to read, but we just could not find anything on the subject of a bilateral replacement.

Mom seemed prepared for and very sure of her surgery. Her legs hurt her so bad, the cortisone shots weren't working anymore (she was getting one in each knee) and it was time to try something new.

Once the decision to have surgery was made, there were several things that needed to be done. Mom's orthopedic surgeon suggested a complete physical examination by her medical or family doctor. This was to ensure that she was in the best possible condition to undergo the operation. Although we did not do the following, you may also want to spend time with the physical therapist who will be managing your rehabilitation after the surgery. The therapist will begin the teaching process before the surgery to ensure that you are ready for the rehabilitation afterwards. One purpose of the pre-operative visit with the physical therapist is to record baseline information. This includes measurements of your current pain levels, what you are able to do, how much swelling you have in the knee, and the amount of movement and strength of each knee. If this is possible, this would be a beneficial thing to do.

A second purpose of the pre-operative visit is to prepare you for surgery. You'll begin practicing some of the exercises you will use right after surgery. You will also be trained in how to use a walker or crutches. Whether or not your surgeon uses a cemented or noncemented type knee prosthesis will determine how much weight you will be able to place on your foot while walking. Lastly, an assessment will be made of any special needs you will have once you return home.

Finally, you may be asked to donate blood before the operation. Blood can be donated 3 to 5 weeks before surgery. Your body will make new blood to replace the donated blood. That way, if you need to have a blood transfusion at the time of surgery, you will receive your own blood.

Mom did decide to donate her own blood for future use, and once she had made the decision to have her knees replaced, she filled out a patient donation request or a physician's order to donate blood form.

There are two types of blood donations—autologous donations and donations directed for the patient by the physician. Autologous donations are when you donate blood for yourself. The patient must be in good health and must meet a minimum red blood cell level. The amount of blood collected depends upon the surgery to be performed. If the patient needs more blood than donated they would receive it from the community blood supply. Mom opted to voluntarily donate her own blood for use after surgery if needed. The surgeon signed the form she would take to the Red Cross.

Mom scheduled her own appointments. The appointment took about an hour for the entire donation process. First, a nurse reviewed her health history, took her blood pressure, temperature and pulse. Then she checked her red blood cell count. She was an acceptable donor, so tags and labels were attached to a bag and the actual blood drawing began. The actual donation took about 10 to 15 minutes. We all wondered how a patient would know if they are receiving their own blood. Often a patient may be alone during this crucial time and how would you be guaranteed that if you needed a transfusion, you would receive your own blood? We were told that autologous, or voluntary blood donations, receive special handling and are kept separate from the community blood supply. Each unit is identified with the patient's name and identification number. Donors receive a receipt, which they must present to the hospital where they are having surgery.

According to mom, donating blood is as easy as pie. I would suspect people who are afraid of needles may have some problem, but mom did not have any problem with things such as that.

In my mom's case you will read that we had to remind each member of her medical team about her blood donations. Although we were told that these donations received special handling and she should not worry about getting her own blood, I must say that if we, her family, were not with her, she would not have received her own blood. It is very important, if not critical, for each patient to have family to oversee the medical procedure and ensure that their loved ones needs are being met.

Shortly before the surgery, some pre-registration forms were sent to mom's home from the hospital. It is important to complete every item on these registration forms and mail them back to the hospital as soon as possible. Most likely your surgery will be scheduled for early morning, and administratively, for the hospital, it is sometimes required that these forms be filled out in advance to avoid any delay the morning of surgery.

On February 12, Mom donated her first pint of blood at the Red Cross in St. Paul. On February 19, a week later, she donated her second pint of blood. On March 3, she had one last appointment with her internist to make sure all was well with her health. Lastly, on March 3, she filled out a living will. This is voluntary for any patient but something you may want to think about. It stated that being of sound mind she willfully and voluntarily made her desire known that her life should not be prolonged under certain conditions that were disclosed on the form.

Chapter Four

The Surgery

The day before mom's surgery, on March 5, she had an appointment with her surgeon for one last visit before the operation. He would give her results of her cardiogram and ask if she had any final questions or concerns about the operation. I am not sure why I decided to go to the doctor with her—up to this point, she had always gone on her own—but this time, I asked if I could go meet the surgeon. I suppose I realized that I wanted to meet her surgeon, the man whose hands we were putting mom's life into. Mom had told me he was wonderful, so if she was happy with him, so was I.

I remember a week or so prior to this mom asked me if we still had a cane. We did; it was an old cane my husband had gotten from his grandfather. We took this with us to the doctor so mom could ask him if it would be ok for her recovery—she had heard she would need one.

She was in really good spirits and did not seem too nervous. We went in to meet with the surgeon. He was a great guy, as mom had said, with a great sense of humor. He said her cardiogram looked great and showed us an x-ray of her knees, which showed us where she had no cartilage left and what was left was bone rubbing against bone. He also brought in a model of what her knee would look like. It was a very large piece of metal. Mom looked a little surprised at that. As stated earlier, in our negligence to ask questions, this was the first we had seen of the appliance that was soon to be mom's knee. She said, "Oh, I didn't know it would be so big and look like that. Since it is metal, will the cold affect it and will I still feel my arthritis?" He confirmed that the cold would affect it. Mom was a little dismayed at this news; I am sure it would have been nice to hear that all of her pain would be gone with the replacement.

It wasn't long after we were in his office that he nonchalantly asked mom, "Well, are we going to do one or both?" We looked at each other with surprise and began to ask some questions. We asked what the recovery time was for both. He said the recovery for a bilateral replacement would be a little more—maybe six months. We asked him to tell us the benefits and shortcomings of both and what he personally thought in my mom's case and after discussing it for a full 5 minutes we looked at each other and shortly thereafter mom said yes. Go for it. In hindsight, we chuckle; such a major decision and we decided it in a mere 5 minutes with one person's opinion.

With the decision made, we then remembered the cane and asked the doctor his advice on that. He said it was much too tall for her. The correct height of a cane can be measured this way: if the person stands up, when they have their hand resting on the curved part of the cane, their elbow should be at a 90 degree angle. Yes, this was too tall. Mom's elbow was probably at a 70 degree angle—bent much too high. We decided we would worry about that later.

Lastly, we asked if she would be "beeped" going through airport security. He said yes but that she would receive a card that allowed her to bypass the security check. Thinking we had all our questions answered, we left the office with no regrets. In fact, it seemed strange but mom seemed like she was anxious to get this over with. Her surgeon had indicated to her that she was in great health and that her attitude was tremendous about surgery—which, apparently, is very important. If a person is apprehensive or worried about these things it affects your mindset.

The night prior to surgery mom was given the following instructions to not eat or drink anything after midnight the day of your surgery. (Later the next day when I stopped at mom's I noticed a note she had written to herself—Do not drink anything!) This was critical because surgery could be canceled if she forgot to follow this instruction. She was also instructed to not wear jewelry, makeup or nail polish the day of surgery. Also, do not bring any valuables with you. Wear casual clothing the day of the surgery. A patient gown will be provided for you and other personal belongings should be brought to the hospital after your surgery. If there is a change in your physical condition between your most recent visit with your surgeon and the day of your surgery, contact your surgeon immediately. Even such minor health conditions as a cold, fever, persistent cough or rash should be reported. A medical history and physical examination must be completed prior to admission. Bring any pre-admission forms or papers your doctor or hospital may have given to you with you to the hospital.

Mom was planning on spending the night at my house, but my daughter had a little cold and mom was afraid she might get sick or infected, so she decided not to. She was already on antibiotics for a slight cold herself. Looking back, I would think it would be a sleepless night for anyone alone the night before major surgery. We picked mom up at 5:35 am. She had a carry bag with a few things—clothes, robe, lipstick, toiletries etc. We went to the hospital and dropped mom off at the front door—a usual occurrence for her these past years with her inability to walk very far—where she would wait for us and we went to park in the hospital parking ramp across the street. We were to go up to 2nd floor surgery. Once there, we filled out some papers and releases—consent for surgery—and verified her insurance. We then took mom to a room where she met a nurse who told her how the morning would go. The nurse took her vitals and during this time, mom mentioned she had just gotten an antibiotic for a little cough. She was a bit concerned about that, but the nurse said it was ok. We mentioned that she had given blood and the nurse was surprised at that. She was not aware of this and apparently her blood donations were not written on her chart, but she said that she would make note of it. She then had mom change into a hospital robe. We stepped outside and took the rest of her stuff with us. From then on, the staff kept her busy. They asked her how her pain was on a scale of one to ten and Mom said about eight or nine—pretty painful. The nurse asked if we had any last minute questions, which we didn't. At that point, our next visitor was her anesthesiologist. He briefly walked her through the procedure. As before, with the nurse, mom told him about her concern with her sore throat and slight cough. His reply was "Well, we don't have to do this, you know. This is purely elective surgery." Which was true, but there was no way we were all going to cancel at this point. Her concern revolved around the fact that she would be lying for 4-6 hours on her back and she was worried about having a coughing attack. She wanted to bring this fact to the attention of one of the doctor's that would be in the operating room. He allayed her fears somewhat, but I think more than that; mom was not about to cancel this surgery. A lot of emotion goes into making this kind of decision and once your mind is made up, a person is ready to go forward. We then talked about the type of anesthesia she would be having.

Anesthesia literally means without pain, and is a medication that is used before an operation to keep the person undergoing the operation from feeling any pain. There are two types of anesthesia that are used in surgery, general and local.

General anesthesia causes the patient to fall asleep during surgery. He or she feels no pain and usually has no memory of the procedure. General anesthesia can be given in a gas through a mask that is placed over the nose and mouth, or it can be injected into a vein.

Local and regional anesthesia causes a small area of the body to become numb, so it won't feel pain, but does not cause the patient to fall asleep. Most local anesthesia is given by injection under the skin. Regional anesthesia is often called spinal, epidural, or nerve block anesthesia. In spinal and epidural anesthesia a drug is injected through a small tube, which is inserted into the base of the back and it blocks all sensation from the lower body. Nerve blocks are an injection of anesthetic around the nerves responsible for feeling in that limb or area of the body.

The type of anesthesia used depends on the type of surgery to be performed. For example, general anesthesia normally is used for major surgeries that involve internal organs. Regional anesthesia is generally used for less complicated operations, such as cesarean childbirth and other procedures done on areas of the body that are below the waist. They can also be used for pain control after a major operation. Local anesthesia is used when suturing cuts or performing dental work.

Sometimes, it is possible to use either general or regional anesthesia for a procedure or operation. Also, the doctor may recommend that a patient be given both types of anesthesia, because when both regional and general anesthesia are used together, less general anesthesia is needed than if general anesthesia if used alone. To decide which type of anesthesia is most appropriate, the risks and benefits of each type used alone or in combination must be carefully considered. In addition, the patient must be sure to tell the doctor of any past allergic reactions to anesthesia.

The benefits of regional anesthesia are that it provides quicker recovery and greater safety because it has fewer side effects and risks.

The benefits of general anesthesia are that the surgeon is able to operate on areas of the body that may be too large to be properly numbed with regional anesthesia and the patient does not remember the surgery.

However, sometimes, when regional anesthesia is used, the patient is given a sedative, which is a drug that causes the patient to relax or fall asleep. Regional anesthesia combined with a sedative may also cause a person not to remember the surgery.

The choice of whether to use general or regional anesthesia or a combination of the two should be thoroughly discussed with your doctor and a decision made jointly based on your individual situation and needs. If the anesthesia will be given by an anesthesiologist, these issues should also be discussed with him or her. An anesthesiologist, as most of you know, is a doctor who specializes in giving anesthesia.

Possible complications of anesthesia may include nausea and vomiting, numbness at the injection site of an anesthetic, headache, sore throat, and mood changes.

More rare complications of anesthesia may include a drop in blood pressure, breathing problems, allergic reactions, inhaling vomit into the lungs, irregular heart beat, cardiac arrest, physical injury, skin inflammation, seizures, permanent brain damage, and death.

Before undergoing anesthesia, you should make sure your doctor knows your complete medical history and avoid eating for twelve hours before the procedure, drinking alcoholic beverages for several days before anesthesia, taking illegal drugs, and also avoid over-the-counter and prescription medications not specifically recommended by the doctor who is performing your surgery or diagnostic procedure, for one day before the surgery or procedure.

Mom's surgeon had not talked about anesthesia at all up to this point. So when the anesthesiologist came in we really did not have any information on which to base our decision. He talked about a spinal and explained it to us. Mom felt she could not be alert for the four hour operation—which would be disturbing to her. We all agreed with this and opted not to continue with a spinal. We mentioned that it was our understanding that she would be unconscious and he said he would speak with the surgeon about her concerns. Shortly thereafter, the surgeon came in. He was wearing his scrubs, which meant that this operation was getting close. He asked her how she was doing, and again asked for any final questions or concerns. A good doctor has a way of calming his patients down and this surgeon exuded an air of confidence and warmth that really helped. We brought up mom's concerns about either a spinal or general anesthesia and subsequently decided on general anesthesia.

About 7:30 a.m. we kissed her good-bye and she was rolled into surgery. We went to a wonderful waiting area where some great computers showed her name and how far along her surgery was. We were told it would be about a 4—6 hour surgery so about 10:30 a.m. or so we decided we would step out for lunch. We stopped and told the volunteer at the desk that we were leaving. They note that fact so that if the doctor comes out while we are gone, he knows that. We went to lunch at a small restaurant around the corner from the hospital and returned about an hour later.

Chapter Five

The Surgical Procedure

Replacing the knee begins with making an incision on the front of the knee to allow access to the knee joint. Once the knee joint is entered, a special cutting tool is placed on the end of the femur. This special tool ensures that the bone is cut keeping the proper alignment to the leg's original angles—even if the arthritis has made you bowlegged or knock-kneed. The upper metal piece of the prosthesis replaces the weight-bearing surfaces of the thighbone and has a groove in which the kneecap moves. The end of the thighbone (femur) is shaped and prepared for the fitting of this metal piece. Several pieces of diseased bone are cut away from the end of the femur so that the artificial knee can be attached. Then, the top of the tibia is cut using another cutting tool that also ensures proper alignment. The undersurface of the kneecap is removed. The lower piece of metal, which will replace the weight-bearing surface of the shinbone, is put in place. It has a plastic surface with a metal backing, which goes down into the shinbone. The top of the shinbone is prepared for the fitting of the metal backing. The femoral component is then fitted on the femur. In the uncemented type of femoral component, the prosthesis is held on the end of the bone because the end of bone has a tapered cut. The metal prosthesis is made to almost exactly match the tapered cut of the bone. Fitting the femoral component onto the end of the bone holds the component in place by friction. In the cemented component, epoxy cement is used to attach the metal prosthesis to the bone. The metal tray that holds the plastic spacer is attached to the end of the tibia. The metal tray is either cemented into place with bone cement, or held in place with screws if the component is the uncemented type. This is not glue but a material that is used to form a bond between the metal and the bone. The screws hold the tray in place until the bone grows into the porous coating. The screws are left in the bone and are not removed. A plastic spacer is attached to the metal tray of the tibial component. If the plastic spacer wears out it can be replaced if the rest of the prosthesis is in good condition—a so-called retread. The patellar button is usually cemented into place behind the patella. The incision is closed, drains are put in, and the post-operative dressing is applied. The incision is down the front of your knee and is approximately 10" long.

Doesn't that sound like a lot of fun? Never fear—you have no idea of what is happening to you. Can you imagine what surgeons can do these days to make our life just a bit easier? My mom's surgeon did a good job!

About 12:40 p.m., the doctor came out and said mom was in recovery. She actually had been out of surgery for about an hour, but he wanted to keep an eye on her and make sure she was going to be ok. He said he wanted to keep her in the Telemetry Unit for a day to watch her heart. He also had her on Morphine for pain and Coumadin, which would promote the thinning of her blood. That was what he was concerned with more than anything—blood clots. I told him she had taken Tylenol like crazy for pain for literally years. Will this Tylenol along with the current blood thinner make her blood too thin? He said no. She would then go to the 8th floor, Orthopedics, tomorrow. He said that in about an hour she would be out of recovery and we could go see her. We then went downstairs to a pay phone to make phone calls—Sue, our sister and mom's third daughter, mom's sister and our sister-in-law who would spread the word to the rest of her children. Her sister did not know she had decided to have both knees done and she did not seem very happy. It was probably best mom had never discussed this with her— she may have been talked out of it.

We went back to the waiting area and watched the computer again. The waiting for the surgery and recovery to be over seems endless. We had been given an idea of how long it would be, but the time dragged on. It helped that we had each other to wait with. Once we talked with the surgeon and Mom was out of recovery we headed to the Telemetry Unit, which was her next stop. We were right outside the room as Mom was being transferred to her bed and we heard her cry out in pain. Then one of the nurses walks out of the room and commented to someone else that she's not sure how she will ever walk again. This was not something we were happy to hear. I winced and looked at my sister, Patty. The nurse came out and said she was sorry we had to hear that. This was the first time I realized exactly how much pain she must be in. The pain must be unbearable.

Chapter Six

Care Immediately Following Surgery

After your operation, there will be a large dressing on your knees with a tensor bandage from your toes to your thigh. A drainage tube attached to a small container will help to remove any blood from the knee joint. This tube will be removed in 1 to 2 days when the drainage has subsided.

Mom had a similar dressing on her knee covering the incision, and she had a tensor bandage on her leg. A draining tube was attached, and we could see the blood draining from that for a few days.

We went into her room once she was moved from the operating bed they rolled her in with to the bed in that room. She was very much disoriented at that point and in tremendous pain. We could see it in her face. She would remain incoherent for the entire day of surgery, which is largely due to the anesthesia and pain medicine she was on. She would mention how thirsty she was, again a result of the anesthesia and was allowed ice chips, which were a big relief to her. She was in quite a bit of pain even though she had a morphine drip attached through an IV. We would talk to Mom when she woke up for short periods of time, but now, almost a year later, she doesn't recall much of that day or the things she herself or any of us talked about. Besides the hemovac tube that drained the blood from the surgical site, she also had an oxygen tube hooked to her nose and an IV in her arm to deliver nourishment, hydration, and antibiotics. The morphine drip mentioned earlier was delivered from a patient-controlled analgesia machine (PCA). The PCA machine was clipped to her gown and the nurse had placed the control unit in her hands. It allowed her to get a dose of painkiller simply by pressing a button. It was programmed to prevent an overdose by only allowing morphine to discharge at prescribed intervals. If she pressed the button too often, she would not get the morphine if it weren't "time" for it. She did not have to worry about this—she could not push this button at all. She was also on Percocet—another major painkiller, Coumadin, a blood thinner and iron. We tried to get her attention during one of her few waking moments to say, "Hi, you made it." That is about how much time we had with her and she went back to sleep. She slept a lot. When she would awaken it would be from the pain and she would tell us groggily how much it hurt. I would push her morphine button for her, which I found out later was a mistake. They wanted her controlling it, not me. If she was not coherent and awake enough to administer her own morphine, no one else should do it for her. No one in the medical field had told me this, so I was unaware of this. She awoke briefly at times throughout the day. She was extremely thirsty! I asked if she could have water and the nurses said no, just ice chips. So we would take turns feeding her ice chips. She was losing a lot of blood. We expressed concern about this and told her nurse once again, (a different nurse) that she had donated two pints of blood, in the event that she would need it. Again, the nurse was not aware of this fact. (We wondered how this could happen. Didn't the morning nurse tell us she would put it on her chart? As I have mentioned, please have a family member present at all times during and after a major operation. You just cannot rely on the patient to be coherent enough to remember anything).

She put it on mom's chart this time—we saw her write it down. She did not need it yet, but that information would be needed in the event that she should need it in the next day or so. Our concern was that if for some reason she needed blood in the middle of the night when no one was present, would the nursing staff know that she was to have her own blood?

She was also attached to a catheter, of course. She would not be up and about for at least a day. About 3:00 p.m. they decided she did need a pint of blood. I asked one more time if they knew she had donated and they said yes. Whew. When the blood was brought in, I confirmed it was hers by the label on the pouch and it was.

When the nurses would leave the room, I would take a look at her chart. Feel free to do this—read anything and every-thing that is available about your family member. This is your right. If the staff makes you feel funny, please persist—those feelings will go away. She also had a white board above her bed that noted her name, medication schedule and Doctor's name. Her chart said she was to be on a liquid diet. We also noticed she was to have specially designed boots on that were to keep the blood from pooling in her legs. Mom had been initially moved to the Telemetry unit so that her heart could be monitored. For this reason, they were not trained in dealing with her orthopedic needs. As a result, she was never hooked up to these "boots" until we reminded them. In fact, if this happens to you or your family member—being held in the heart unit or maybe even intensive care, remember that they are not trained in orthopedics and may need reminding of certain procedures. Granted this is not our job to administer the care, but our experience was that we had to ask lots of questions, even if it made the staff uncomfortable or angry with you, because they changed shifts frequently and not all information was passed along to each nurse. Once again, this is why we are writing this book—I hope it helps someone in the future. We went into this blind, but sure learned a lot!

I stayed with her until 6 p.m. and Patty decided she would stay with her for the duration. We were worried about her blood pressure which was about 80/50, again a normal occurrence for postoperative surgery, but although normal, something to keep watch of. Blood pressure can drop to dangerous levels if not monitored correctly we were told. I came back about 8 p.m. and Patty was still there. Mike, our brother, also visited that evening. Mom was still very much out of it. She was in a very lethargic state. She would wake up from a deep sleep and turn to us and say something that sometimes made no sense at all and at other times would fit entirely into our discussion. We never really knew if she was aware of what was going on around her or not. We knew, though, that this was a result of all of the strong medication she was on. We both stayed until 10 p.m. Neither of us wanted to go, but we were so tired. We decided to talk to the nurses and see exactly how they monitored her. Maybe if we felt like she was in good hands, we would feel better going home. They each had a monitor like TV screen that they could monitor each patient's heartbeat. We asked if she had her own nurse, which she did, and after a few more questions, we felt a little more comfortable about leaving her, so we did. My concern, as that first day wore on, was her blood pressure. I knew it wouldn't be normal for a while after surgery, but hers seemed awfully low to me. It had, though, stabilized over the past few hours, so eventually we went home for the night.

Chapter Seven

Day 2

Patty called the hospital right away that first morning after surgery. Her main concern was if Mom had a restful night and how was her blood pressure? She was told it had gone down to 85/18. I received a call from Patty about 7:00 a.m. I had gotten up early and was planning on going to the hospital so I was already awake. Patty said she had called the hospital to see how she had done overnight and they said her BP had dropped to 85/18. I panicked. Patty wanted to know when I was going in and I said right away—I was on my way. I sped (literally) to the hospital. I met with her nurse, in her room and she told me that the lowest her blood pressure had gotten all night was 85/53 and that we were misinformed. Again, how can some of these things happen? It was like a ton of weight was lifted off of my shoulders, and although I was very angry about the miscommunication, it just didn't matter anymore. I stepped in to see mom. She was awake and looked amazingly good for just having a bilateral knee replacement. In fact I thought she looked better than I ever imagined. We talked a little and she mentioned to me that the doctor was there. I said, the surgeon? She replied, no, her regular doctor, whom I had never met. I went out to introduce myself to him and speak with him about her condition. He confirmed her blood pressure was still about 80 over 50. This was low, but understandable for post surgery. He thought she was doing absolutely great and did not really have too much to add. We only spent a minute or two talking. I went back in and mom and I talked a little more. She was in good spirits and slightly coherent, but tired. Shortly afterward her breakfast came, which was pancakes and orange juice. She said she was so thirsty so I gave her some of her orange juice. She immediately got nauseous and said she felt like she was going to vomit, but didn't. She thought maybe she would try a bite of pancakes—which might help, although she was not hungry at all. (Remember how I previously mentioned that the family members should be aware of everything? I had not noticed the white board above her bed that noted a liquid diet or I would have said something to the people bringing her breakfast. That was our mistake. This is what we hope to bring to your attention, so the same does not happen to you.) At that moment the surgeon came in and said, "What are you eating?" She, of course, answered "pancakes". He wanted to know who had given her pancakes—she was not supposed to have anything to eat at all—she was supposed to be on a liquid diet. He was livid. Again, I am reluctant to say too much, but so much responsibility is on the patient's and family's shoulders as far as care goes. It is just so important to be asking questions, ensuring that if the patient is supposed to be on a liquid diet, that they are, that if they donate blood, they receive it, etc.

Her surgeon spent quite a bit of time with her and mom seemed very glad to see that he thought her progress was so good. He told her she was doing great. (Later we found out that he reprimanded the nurses for the care of his patient—another sign of a good doctor.) Before he left, he told mom and me that she could have as much pain medication as she wanted—we should just ask. He also said she would probably move to the orthopedic floor that day. Indeed, about 9:00 a.m., they moved her to the 8th floor. This was difficult and very painful! Once there she went to a temporary room until her primary room was ready. Another patient was not quite out of her permanent room, so she would have to make another move in a few hours.

Here on the orthopedic floor, she got a nurse who she loved. He was very gentle and seemed to know what he was doing. He told her they were going to get her hooked up that day to something called a CPM machine. CPM or continuous passive motion was a machine that would move her knees alternately for her.

Continuous Passive Motion (CPM) is a postoperative treatment method that is designed to aid recovery after joint surgery. In most patients after extensive joint surgery, attempts at joint motion cause pain and as a result, the patient fails to move the joint. This allows the tissue around the joint to become stiff and for scar tissue to form resulting in a joint which has limited range of motion and often may take months of physical therapy to recover that motion. Passive range of motion means that the joint is moved without the patient's muscles being used. Continuous Passive Motion devices are machines that have been developed for patients to use after surgery. Applied post-operatively, this device may be used on an inpatient or an outpatient basis. By using a motorized device to very gradually move the joint, it is possible to significantly accelerate recovery time by decreasing soft tissue stiffness, increasing range of motion, promoting healing of joint surfaces and soft tissue, and preventing the development of motion-limiting adhesions (scar tissue). Interestingly, this is accomplished without patient effort (passively) as the machine moves a joint through a defined, prescribed range of motion for an extended period of time. Even more surprisingly, studies have shown that patients using CPM devices require less pain medication then patients who have had the same type of surgery and are not using this device. The physician prescribes how the CPM unit should be used by the patient (speed, duration of usage, amount of motion, rate of increase of motion, etc.). Once the device is setup and in use by the patient, the nurse regularly follows up with the patient to ensure that the patient is comfortable, that the equipment is functioning properly, that the patient is using the equipment properly and that all questions are answered. This device was very beneficial for mom's recovery, because it helped keep her knee limber and keep scar tissue from forming.

By the time Patty and her husband, Marty got to the hospital, Mom had been moved to this temporary room on the

8th floor while her permanent room was being prepared. Mom was still very much "in and out of it". Right before she was moved to the permanent room a physical therapist and an assistant came in. The therapist asked questions about Patty's home (where Mom would stay for a while before she went home by herself), the number of steps in her house, etc. He also asked about the number of steps in mom's home.

Mom was started on the CPM machines immediately. The therapist would return later that day to have her sit up. She did ask if the same therapist would return the next day but was told no, which was too bad, because she really liked him. This seemed the case with the nurses as well as the PT's. Mom rarely saw the same person(s) for more than one shift during her hospital stay. Lots of times we wondered if the nurses wrote everything on Mom's chart and when one shift ended, did the new nurse look at the chart? We, her family, seemed to be telling the nurses things it seemed they should know. We realized they had more than one patient, but it seems they should have been more informed. There seemed to be no two people who adjusted the CPM machines the same. This continued at the Transitional Care Unit center also. No one really seemed to know for sure how to position

Mom's legs in the CPM's, or what degree they should be set at or for how long. Mom let them know when a machine was set too high or too fast, and she did feel tremendous relief when they were on. She said it felt very good. She had the CPM machines alternated on her knees and they gently flexed her knees at varying degrees. It was set at very small degrees at first and increased gradually each time.

Mom was becoming a lot more coherent by the afternoon of this day, and when I returned she was moved once more to her permanent room across the way.

To be noted, immediately after waking up and for several days after surgery, breathing and circulation exercises are important. Inactivity following surgery allows secretions to collect in the lungs. These secretions are a good breeding ground for germs, which can cause pneumonia. Deep breathing and coughing to move secretions out of the lungs can decrease this risk.

Mom was given a small unit that she was to inhale into to keep her lungs clear. It was a small plastic unit that had a hose attached to it. When you inhale on this hose it brings a small disc up the tube by varying degrees depending on the patients force of inhalation. The nurses told mom she should have that disc go to 10 which is the maximum. Her first try, she could barely get it to two. We had her do it a couple more times, but it wore her out. As the days went on, although this unit sat on her table right in front of her, we had to remind her to use it whenever we were there. She just did not remember. Her state of mind was such that she was just getting by day by day. There seemed to be so much for her to remember. We knew that if we were not there keeping an eye on her, the staff probably would not have the time to do it. For this reason, Patty and I made sure that if we were not there, one of our brothers was.

Other diaphragmatic breathing exercises might include doing the following. While in a lying or sitting position, take a breath in until your lungs are almost full. Without breathing out, "top up" your lungs with 3 sniffs in through your nose. Hold your breath for 5 seconds, and then breathe out. Repeat 6 times every hour you are awake.

With inactivity, your circulation slows down. When this happens, you are prone to developing more swelling in your operated leg and are at risk of developing blood clots, which can be very serious. Frequent muscle pumping and early walking will help decrease the swelling and the risk of developing a blood clot. Some exercises to keep your blood circulating include:

Ankle Pumping—Increase your circulation by pointing your toes downward, then up, in a slow steady motion. Repeat 20 times every hour you are awake.

Quadriceps Sets—This is an isometric exercise: there is no movement involved. Tighten the quadriceps muscles by pressing your knee down into the bed. Hold for 5 seconds. Relax. Repeat 10 times every hour you are awake.

Gluteal Sets—While lying down on your back, squeeze your buttocks together. Hold tightly for 5 seconds. Relax. Repeat 10 times every hour you are awake.

Chapter Eight

Day 3

When appropriate with your healing process, while you are in the hospital it is important that you start a regimen of range of motion exercises walking and exercises for strength and flexibility. The physical therapist will schedule your first visit soon after surgery. Therapy will focus on the range of motion in the knee. Gentle movement will be used to help you begin bending and straightening of the knee. Next, you'll go over your exercise regimen. When you are stabilized, your therapist will assist you up for a short walk using crutches or a walker. Physical therapy will continue once or twice a day. You will be on your way home when you can safely get into and out of bed, walk up to 75 feet with crutches or a walker, go up and down a flight of stairs, and get to the bathroom.

This particular morning, her nurse talked about therapy and the fact that they would get her walking maybe that day or the next at the latest. This seemed unfathomable to mom. She could absolutely not imagine bearing down on her knees in the near future at all. In the end, she did not have any walking therapy in the hospital—therapy started when she went to the rehabilitation home. After your operation, the goal of the therapist is to prepare you for discharge by helping you achieve independence as safely and quickly as possible.

Bending and straightening of the knee begins as soon as possible after surgery with the assistance of the physical therapist. 70—90 degrees of bending is the goal before you go home. This may be painful but must be done in order to achieve your goals. It will not cause any damage to your incision or the joint replacement.

Within 2 to 3 days, you will begin to walk with a walker or crutches. You will be taught how to climb stairs before you go home.

Today was going to be her first day with a physical therapist. They wanted to get her to stand and possibly sit on the commode. Mom had some concerns about the therapist. First of all, she was concerned that the she was very small and would not be able to help her up. What the therapist did to alleviate mom's fears was to have a nurse help her. The first thing they needed to do was to get mom sitting up. Remember she has been lying down for 2 days. When she got up (with 100% help from the therapist and nurse) she had to sit for a minute or two. She was extremely dizzy. They told her that their goal was to have her slide forward on the bed and have her stand. There was one of them on each side of her to hold her up and she was not going to fall forward. If she fell back, she would land on the bed. No problem, right? Her knees and legs were put in leg immobilizers so that she could not bend them. They got mom on her feet for a few seconds, but no longer than that. As time went on this increased, but in mom's case it was first a few seconds, then a minute, then longer etc. The goal was to get her on the commode that day, but it was not going to happen. Mom was not physically able to do it. As mentioned before, Mom saw several different PT's at the hospital. Mom's arms were fairly weak so she couldn't push herself up very well. I believe she saw a PT twice a day in the hospital and with each visit she was able to do a little more.

Mom had no appetite but we filled out her menus anyway. She was pretty emotional, which is normal, I think. We knew she needed to eat to keep up her strength. Sue, our younger sister, had told her that quite a few times. Also, her fluid intake and outgo were monitored (she continued with the bedpan since she wasn't able to walk to the toilet yet) so she was encouraged by the nursing staff to eat if at all possible as well.

As a side note, ice packs can be applied around the knee joint to help reduce swelling and pain. Some swelling and pain is normal. Ice, elevation, and a balance of rest and activity can control this. Mom used lots of ice packs now and for weeks after—they felt great!

That day a representative from the insurance company came in and talked about where she was going to go after her stay at the hospital. Some patients are able to go home, but for the majority of patients, they really should go to a rehabilitation center for a week before they go home and try to function on their own. There were two choices for mom—one was closer than the other and smaller, so that was the one that was chosen.

About 9 a.m. that day, during one of her wakeful periods, I asked her how she was feeling. She said she felt a little funny. I asked what she meant and she could not describe it, just funny. I told the nurse the next time she was in the room, and the nurse asked if she felt like she might need something to calm down. I asked if she felt a little jittery or anxious and she said yes. They told me they would bring her some Ativan. It finally came at 1:00 p.m.—four hours later! I suppose they needed to call the doctor and leave a message and get his approval. I can understand that, but it was a good thing we weren't asking for pain medication.

I stayed until our brother, Jim, came to visit. During the time he was visiting, mom noticed that her arm was starting to hurt. I think she had so much going on those first few days that nothing really registered. But this she was aware of. She was hooked up to so many things and still slightly out of it, that if she knew her arm was hurting, I am sure it was! My brother looked her over and noticed that the needle in her arm that was providing saline to her system had slipped out and the saline was draining directly into her arm. She got extremely scared. My brother called the nurses and in the process of trying to hook her up again, they could not find a vein. (A usual occurrence for her). She had what turned out to be a mild panic attack. She got very scared that the needle had dislodged. Remember that your family member has gone through a major surgery, are in tremendous pain and are going through an emotional recovery. It is so important that you are there to help in any way you can. I arrived back at the hospital right about when things were starting to calm down. She looked good, had regained her composure and seemed in pretty good spirits.

Chapter Nine

The Last Days in the Hospital

The next few days some exciting things happened which told us that mom was really on the road to recovery. On her third day in the hospital the surgeon said he wanted to "unhook" her from everything except her oxygen. He was still a little concerned about her oxygen. We decided to have her stay on that for another day and decided that she needed to concentrate on her inhaling into her little machine to help her lungs. But what a joy it was for her to have all those needles removed. It had been really bothering her—she felt so trapped!

I believe it was the next day that the nurses removed her bandages and we got our first look at the incision. What an incision! The cut on her left knee was longer that the one on the right. We wondered aloud why that was. We would ask. Mom felt she always had someone in the room wanting to do something to or for her, and so she only got catnaps during the day, which can be frustrating. I think her nights were restful, though.

The last day at the hospital was no different. She was kept busy until it was time to be taken to the TCU—Transitional Care Unit. Patty and our sister in law, Bonnie, went to the hospital and packed up all her belongings. A van then took her—HMO transportation—to the center. The young driver seemed very nice. This was best; they were equipped to transport her in her wheelchair, with her legs straight out. Remember you might be in immobilizers for a period of time while your knees are healing. It is too painful for them to be moved on our own—the CPM machine did any movement that is prescribed this early on. One thing the van driver wondered aloud to mom when they got to the TCU, was why there were no wheelchair accessible doors? All these are little things for you to consider and look into prior to surgery if possible.

The nurses at the rehab center spent hours getting mom settled—it was a busy day. When she got there she received information about her phone extension, bathing, meal times, visiting hours etc. I visited her that evening and found out they also had her doing therapy that first day. Wow, it is true; the patient should be moving quickly. She settled in early that night, exhausted.

Chapter Ten

Rehabilitation

Depending on the patient, the surgeon, and the individual time of recovery, there may be a need to have the patient go to a rehabilitation center for another week after surgery, which was my mom's case. The average length of stay in the hospital following a total knee replacement is about seven days. Some people go directly home on discharge and manage very well. But, not all patients are ready to go home to a relative's house quite yet. The rehab center is generally so much more equipped to handle a recovering knee patient—they have the appliances a knee patient needs, wheelchairs, ramps, adjustable beds etc. In my mom's case, although she wanted to go home to my sister's, she just couldn't. She had very serious knee surgery and it really was not an option for her—it was required that she go to a rehabilitation center for another week.

The next day Patty visited for a short while. She had lunch with her while she was there. Mom's appetite was slowly coming back. She had a sponge bath and since she had bed-sores, had powder put on her behind. She had her bedding changed and a short while after that got to get dressed in something other than a hospital gown for the first time. She leaned against the bed then put on her shorts with the help of a long pair of tongs—an appliance that would help her grab garments and pull them on. Once her blouse was on she was wheeled down to physical therapy. During her stay at the TCU I only watched her do some of her exercises once.

The second day at the rehab center, our sister, Sue, from Texas came into town for a week. She would share in the visits and stay with Patty and her family when mom was finally transferred to a home setting.

That morning Sue and I went to see mom early. We went by her house first and picked up some things she wanted. She wanted her mail, some clean clothes, etc. When we arrived, she was sitting up in her wheel chair facing the window waiting for us. What an amazing sight. She had the leg pieces on the wheel chair positioned such that her legs were straight out from the chair, keeping the knees straight. She was very happy to see us! We visited for a while. She read her mail and was pleased to see a lot of other get-well cards. We visited for much of the day. Early evening, Sue packed up her dirty laundry to go home. She was staying at Jim and his wife Kari's house—he had a car she would be able to use for the week. Sue stayed for rehab that day and she had a very nice nurse. She was very patient and seemed to make the experience less traumatic with her kindness.

With Sue in town, she took over most of the patient watch. Usually by the time she got out there each day, mom had had breakfast and was on the way to morning rehab. The goal was to get her out of rehab and to be able to maneuver stairs (since she has 2 sets of them in her house), and to be able to bend the knee to 90 degrees. This never ceases to amaze mom because she says that she has not been able to bend her knees to 90 degrees normally for as long as she can remember. One nurse really pressured mom to move fast at the rehab. I know that mom was anxious to get out of the rehab facility, and was very vocal about it, but this nurse obviously wanted to help her to get out of there! There were several exercises she had at each rehab session. She had to lie on a mat and put her leg on a board. She had a slick bootie on and a towel around her foot. She would hold the ends of the towel and pull them to flex her knees. She had one exercise where she put her knee over a padded coffee can and had to extend the leg up from a bent position. Over time, she went from being wheeled to the rehab mat, to being wheeled to the rehab room and made to walk to the mat, to having to walk with her walker all the way from her room. Walking seemed to be easy for her—almost therapeutic. When she got stiff or sore, she would get up and walk around with her walker. Stairs were also amazingly easy for her. One would think that after knee surgery stairs would be tough, but it appeared that movement itself was much easier than being stagnant. That would continue to be the case during home therapy and seems to still be the case now. On good days, she can sit through a movie, but on bad days, she can't.

Something to note is that although this was a rehabilitation center, we were getting slightly frustrated. We would turn on mom's call light for pain medication and wait for 45 minutes to an hour. They would never come unless we went out to the hallway and got someone. Mom also sat for two nights in urine stained sheets before anyone changed her. It is so important to possibly visit the center you have in mind, and again, do as much homework as you can before you place a loved one in someone else's care. In hindsight, the rehab center was probably not the best choice of facilities, but who knew at the time of making the decision. That is one thing I would highly recommend looking into prior to the surgery. Ask well in advance what the choices would be and then go visit them prior to rehab. This center seemed to cater more to geriatric care rather than orthopedic rehabilitation. They were frequently late with meals, pain medication, and therapy and they seemed to greatly resent suggestions that they were not punctual. Sadly enough, we would not recommend that a person receiving rehab be left alone for any length of time.

I don't know if the recovery time for all patients with bilateral knee replacement is the same, but I sure thought that the time from surgery to walking to being able to climb stairs was remarkable in mom's case. I was amazed that they could go in and totally replace her knees and she could be walking (even with a walker) and taking stairs within 2 weeks! I realize that this does not constitute the entire recovery period (which appears to be more like 9-12 months), but I thought this initial 2 weeks was amazing! About her 5th or 6th day at the TCU she walked (with a walker) all the way back to the room.

Part of her rehab also included afternoon sessions with the occupational therapist. This woman helped mom figure out things like using a walker in a kitchen, how to get things out of the refrigerator while using a walker, how to safely use kitchen appliances while using a walker, etc. These are all things I never thought about before. They seemed a little remedial, but once you are dependent on a walker to stabilize and balance your body, letting go with one hand to do things around the house might be a little scary. Mom was bored with it, but it was important to do just the same.

Her third day there, a van came and was to take us to see the surgeon. Mom took her walker with her but we took her in her wheelchair. The nurse took out her staples and said that the incision looked good. The surgeon came in and was a little surprised to see her in a wheelchair. He said that if she could use her walker, then get out of the chair! She did as soon as we got back to the rehab center! The surgeon said the incision looked good. I got to meet him and thought he was very nice as well. He took out the models and showed me what the prostheses looked like. Very impressive little hunk of metal I must say! He thought she was progressing fine and said when she met all of the rehab requirements of the rehab center that she could go home.

This is a day to remember, because this is the day Mom finally got a shower in the center. It must feel terribly gross to not have a shower for a week. The things we take for granted!

Chapter Eleven

Going Home

On March 18, 12 days after surgery, mom was discharged from the rehab center. She was given instructions to wear TED stockings 24 hours a day and use knee immobilizers when walking. She was also told to see her primary doctor 2 days after discharge for a blood test on Friday. Her "home care" would start on March 20th. She was deemed independent by the rehab center on the following items: bed mobility, toileting, hygiene/grooming, eating, and meal preparation. The following comments were made though—they recommended a raised toilet seat or over the toilet commode. They also recommended supervision initially while bathing. Recommended for the tub was a tub seat with a back, or you could also consider a grab rail for edge of tub. She was to have assistance with dishes, dusting and bed making and must obtain approval from her surgeon prior to resuming driving. Also, she was to have exercises at home every day and she was to have outpatient physical therapy three times a week for three weeks.

Almost 2 weeks after the surgery (3/19) Mom went to a place she could safely call home to do some recuperating, Patty's house. There was no way she was ready to be on her own yet. She was happy to see her kitty, Chelsea and vice versa. We got her settled in to her temporary bedroom. She was very chilled in this room. This could have been due to the fact that her blood was redirected to healing her knees and away from her peripheral areas; we would have to check with her doctors about this, but with most post-op orthopedic patients, external sources of heat are very important. We got her all settled in at Patty's, and it seemed one milestone had been reached.

Once Mom was settled in, Sue made some calls and we found a place locally to get Mom an adjustable chair for the shower and a raised toilet seat. Sue also got her some strap on hot/cool pads from a drug store. They are stretchy with Velcro so she could put them on while she slept. She liked to keep ice on her knees, as that made them feel better. She kept ice on almost constantly at first. It would be interesting to find out from the surgeon though if this was good, as most sports rehabbers would tell you not to keep ice on for more than 30 minutes at a time.

She already had a walker. Insurance pays for all or most of the walker but the patient pays for any additional supplies. It's worth it though; Mom got lots of use out of the seat and the chair. She couldn't have done it without them! Things were starting to heal, as evidenced by the patient feeling a lot of pain, so the packs were a big relief to Mom.

One thing we had not thought of and we discovered was very difficult for mom, was getting into and out of bed. The height was just high enough to make it difficult for her. What we did was position a "step" such as the ones used in exercise regimens just to the side of the bed. This gave her just enough height to get in. She did not have to bend her knee very much to step onto the stepper, and once she was on the step, she could kind of move her bottom around and slide into bed. We forget, she cannot bend her knees and it is amazing how much a person bends their knees in the course of ordinary life that we don't even realize.

She felt pretty good being out of the rehab center. Her daily routine involved going through her mail, sorting laundry and spending time with Chelsea. Then it was time for a nap. She was on a pretty rigorous medication schedule, so she slept a lot and Sue woke her up for pill time. She did lots of leg exercises and walked around a lot at Patty's house. Sue was able to stay for 2 nights so she took the pill-giving duty. As she said, Mom was on a variety of medications and it was important she did not miss taking anything.

Sue slept downstairs and had an alarm set for the middle of the night and the early morning medications. The Coumadin (the medication to prevent blood clots) was very important to be given on a regular basis. After major orthopedic surgery, the potential for blood to pool and form clots in immobile limbs is great and these clots could enter the venous system and cause an embolus, which could travel to the heart or to the lungs. This is a very serious condition and was the last thing the people at the rehab center told us when we left. They said that if she ever felt short of breath, had trouble breathing, or had a sharp pain or a sensation of heat in one of her legs, that this was a medical emergency and to call 911 immediately.

On Friday, we had to make the long trek to have her Coumadin levels checked at the clinic. When we got there, I called the home rehab facility to arrange for a nurse to go out to Patty's house 3 times a week. They said that we would have someone out at 1:00 p.m. I didn't think we could get there in time, but they highly recommended trying, as the person they wanted to send out was not available if we didn't start him that day. I agreed and mom was very upset because she was not emotionally ready to start with the rehab all over again. This stress combined with the fact that the nurse at the clinic would not listen to mom caused her to break down crying while we were getting her blood drawn. She said she was fine; she just wanted them to find a vein and get the blood. The nurse could not find a vein and mom said, "I know there is a vein right here, it doesn't look like it, but if you just put the needle straight down, you will get blood. I swear!" The nurse didn't believe her, treated her like a pincushion and when mom started crying, she felt bad, followed directions, and lo and behold, got blood! We rushed home and just barely beat the nurse to Patty's house.

The therapist came for the first time the day after Mom got out of the hospital. She was pretty tired most of the time and dreaded his coming at first. Before he left he set days and times when he would come back. He was very nice and answered all her questions. He first watched her on the walker, checked to see what she could do and then explained what he was going to do. Mom really liked it once he was here and working with her. Patty's husband, Marty, had a cane that the therapist measured and we cut it for her future use. Mom spent most of her days resting, reading, catching up on paperwork or watching TV. Each day it seemed as if she spent less time in bed and was up and walking.

Once you are at home, the physical therapist will likely come to your home for treatment. This is to ensure you are safe in and around your home. Your therapist will probably see you for at least one safety check visit and to go over your exercise program again. You may need as many as three visits at home before beginning outpatient physical therapy.

The at-home therapist I had was absolutely great. (I, the patient, will begin to interject my thoughts here—I am starting to feel good and can remember much of what is now happening.) He told me that he had taken care of many bilateral patients, so I knew I was in good hands. Each time he came—twice a week for two weeks—he pushed my legs a bit further—apparently they like you to be at a particular level before he leaves you completely. I, at first, felt he was pushing too hard, but as time progressed I felt his pushing me to excel was just what a person needs to move onward and upward. I used pressure stockings all the time—day and night—until the surgeon finally told me I could remove them—which was several weeks later.

Once you begin outpatient physical therapy, several key areas will be addressed. Your therapist may choose one or more treatments, such as heat, ice, or electrical stimulation, to help reduce any persistent swelling or pain. Continue to use your walker or crutches. If you had a cemented prosthesis, you can increase the amount of weight you place on your sore leg(s) until you feel uncomfortable. If you had a noncemented prosthesis, place only your toes down until your doctor or therapist allows you to increase the amount of weight you can bear.

Range of motion exercises will help you regain full bending and straightening of your knee. Your exercise program will include strengthening, balance, endurance, and functional activities. Your strengthening program will focus on key muscle groups in the buttocks and hips, thigh, and calf muscles. When you are allowed full weight bearing, several balance exercises will be used to further stabilize your knee. Endurance can be achieved by riding a stationary bike, swimming laps, and using an upper body ergometer (upper cycle). Finally, you will be taught a special group of exercises that simulate your day-to-day activities, like going up and down steps, squatting, raising up on your toes, and bending down. Later, specific exercises may be chosen to simulate the physical demands of your work or hobby.

Emphasis continues to be on gaining movement, both bending and straightening, improving the strength of the thigh muscles, and improving walking. It is good to go for a walk everyday. In good weather when sidewalks are free of ice, walk outside. In poor weather, walk in the hallway of an apartment building or in a shopping mall when it's not busy.

Your knee will continue to be warm and swollen for several weeks following surgery, and variable discomfort will be present. This is quite normal as the healing process continues. Ice packs may be applied regularly to help reduce pain and swelling. If swelling is a problem, sitting should be limited to short periods.

The therapist will help you to progress your exercises, as you are able. Do the exercises prescribed for you regularly and gradually increase the frequency and distance of your walks using your walker or crutches.

Sue had one more night with the alarm clock and medications, and then it was Saturday morning and she had to go home.

Chapter Twelve

Complications

As with all major surgical procedures, complications can occur. The most common complications following knee replacement are thrombophlebitis (blood clots), infection in the joint, stiffness of the joint and loosening of the joint. This is not intended to be a complete list of the possible complications, but these are the most common.

Thrombophlebitis, sometimes called Deep Venous Thrombosis (DVT), can occur after any operation. It is more likely to occur following surgery on the hip, pelvis, or knee. DVT occurs when the blood in the large veins of the leg forms blood clots within the veins. This may cause the leg to swell and become warm to the touch and painful. If the blood clots in the veins break apart they can travel to the lung. Once in the lung they get lodged in the capillaries of the lung and cut off the blood supply to a portion of the lung. This is called a pulmonary embolism. Pulmonary means "lung". An embolism is a fragment of something traveling through the vascular system. Most surgeons take preventing DVT very seriously. There are many ways to reduce the risk of DVT, but probably the most effective is getting you moving around as soon as possible!

Some of the commonly used preventative measures include pressure stockings to keep the blood in the legs moving and medications that thin the blood and prevent blood clots from forming.

Infection can be a very serious complication following an artificial joint. The chance of getting an infection following total knee replacement is probably around 1 in 100 replacements. Some infections may show up very early—before you leave the hospital. Others may not show up for months, or even years, after the operation. Also, an infection can spread into the artificial joint from other infected areas. I now understand that for the rest of my life I must take antibiotics before any surgery or dental work because of the possibility of infection. If a person does get infection in the prosthesis it is a very difficult thing to get rid of—with the possibility of surgery once more to get rid of that infection. My feeling about this is that I surely will take the antibiotics to rid myself of any chance of getting an infection. That is not what I want after a year of recuperation.

In some cases, the ability to bend the knee does not return to normal after an artificial knee replacement. As mentioned earlier, many orthopedic surgeons are now using a machine known as a CPM machine (Constant Passive Motion) immediately after surgery to try and increase the range of motion following artificial knee replacement. Other orthopedic surgeons rely on physical therapy beginning immediately after the surgery to regain the motion. It is not clear which is the best approach. As mentioned earlier, I used the CPM machine almost immediately after surgery and I thought it was great. You put your legs in this machine and it moves your leg—back and forth—bending it a little more each time you use the machine. My surgeon was one of those surgeons who liked that approach. Both approaches have benefits and risks, and the surgeon based on his experience and preferences usually makes the choice.

To be able to use the leg effectively to rise from a chair, the knee must bend at least to 90 degrees. A desirable range of motion should be greater than 110 degrees. Balancing of the ligaments and soft tissues (during surgery) is the most important determining factor in regaining an adequate range of motion following knee replacement, but sometimes increased scarring after surgery can lead to an increasingly stiff knee. I am able to use my legs effectively today due to the fact that I am regularly climbing stairs, walking and exercising my legs when I go to bed. I am an active person, and still work for a living and I would not be able to be one of these people who would sit back and wait for things to happen without trying to make them happen. If this occurs, your surgeon may recommend taking you back to the operating room, placing you under anesthesia once again, and forcefully manipulating the knee to regain motion. Basically, this allows the surgeon to break up and stretch the scar tissue without you feeling it. The goal is to increase the motion in the knee without injuring the joint

The major reason that artificial joints eventually fail continues to be loosening of the joint where the metal or cement meets the bone. There have been great advances in extending the life of an artificial joint. Still, most joints will eventually loosen and require a revision. Hopefully, you can expect 12-15 years of service from your artificial knee. In some cases the knee will loosen earlier than that. Just like your diseased knee, a loose joint causes pain. Once the pain becomes unbearable, another operation will probably be required to replace the knee.

Please remember, it is important to continue the exercise program given to you by your physical therapist as part of your daily routine. Gradually increase your level of activity by adding different activities into your routine. Remember —your endurance will continue to improve for several months. Avoid any sudden jarring or twisting activity of the knee. You will usually see your surgeon about 6 to 8 weeks following surgery for review. If you are having surgery or dental work in the future, inform the doctor that you have a joint replacement. You will need to take an antibiotic prior to any intrusive surgery.

In a small percentage of people, problems develop that require medical attention. Blood clots may develop in the lower leg following surgery and decreased activity. Infection can occur around the replacement in approximately 1% of people following knee surgery. Antibiotic therapy would be required and further surgery is occasionally necessary. Loosening of one of the components over time occasionally occurs and may relate to excessive stress on the joint. Contact your surgeon or family doctor if any problems concern you (i.e. swelling, redness, and/or warmth).

In our case, mom recovered slowly. About a week after she was released from the rehab center, Patty got her out of the house for a BP check. While she was there she also had the Doctor check her legs—she was concerned because her ankles were so swollen. Just to be on the safe side, he decided to have an ultrasound done. We took her back to the same hospital—if that wasn't a mixture of emotions, I don't know what was. We put her in a wheelchair and went to admitting. They had us fill out some forms and had us go to the x-ray unit. We waited a little while and then were called in. Mom said she wanted me to go with. Once in the room, the technician who was extremely nice had her get her shorts off. I helped her—it was very hard for her—almost impossible, and had her take off her TED's stocking which she had been wearing since day two. The technician left the room and mom started crying. It had scared the heck out of her—she was thinking that after going through all that surgery—now to have something serious happen like a blood clot. If she went through all of this for a blood clot she didn't know what she would do. After much probing, mom asked how everything looked. She said, "I'm smiling, and that is good news." Everything was ok. In fact, one thing she learned while she was there was that she had a Baker's cyst behind her left knee, which bothers her to this day. We went back home but on the way she had me stop at the grocery store. My mom was having trouble with her bowel movements and she wanted to get an enema, chocolate and suppositories. She was on iron and still had not had a bowel movement and was getting very uncomfortable. (This is common —the drugs you are given during major operations, shut down all your internal functions for obvious reasons, and then if you are taking Iron for your blood, things can get very backed up!)

After Sue left Patty took over the middle of the night ice pack and pill giving duty. After about 2 weeks when Patty was waking mom up to take her pain pills she suggested we leave ice packs in a cooler so she could change her own. She also left the alarm clock to wake her to take her pills. Mom had an outing on April 5th, my brother Tom's birthday. She spent the afternoon with him and his family and was very glad to get out of the house.

Chapter Thirteen

On My Own

Easter was April 12th. Patty made a ham and all the fixings and after we ate they took mom and Chelsea, mom's cat home. She hadn't been back for 38 days and had told us this day was her goal to be on her own! They stayed awhile and tried to get everything ready for her. It was a time of mixed emotions for her, we were sure. After over a month of being dependent on someone for a lot of things she's all of a sudden on her own. Marty loaned her a hip pack to carry her cell phone around in. That way if anything happened she'd be able to call someone to help. Fortunately she never needed to use it.

A couple days later, mom came to my house for a shower. She still could not do a lot on her own. Although she was slowly trying to gain her independence, there were some things such as showering that just were not safe for her to do. She wore slippers in the shower to avoid slipping—the kind with the rubber bottoms. I helped her in the shower and when she was done she sat on the couch and looked like a new person. She said it had never felt so good to have a shower.

I stopped over one night a few days later. It was a bad night. She needed to fend for herself and things were just so much harder than she thought they would be. I took her ice packs up to her bedroom for her and tried to help in any other ways she needed. Just as we leaving, she told me about how her left knee seemed to pop as she got up. We talked about how much pain she was still in and all of a sudden she broke down crying. She said she was so tired of being in pain. Years of arthritis and now this. I felt terrible for her, but she said she would be fine. I asked if I should stay but she said no. She knew she had to do this, but was not prepared for the emotions that were now setting in. What she once thought would be a quick recovery, was turning into months, and although her surgeon had said six months to a year, she just did not want to believe this. I got her upstairs and she fell into bed. I positioned a towel under her knees and she lay back, drained physically and emotionally.

I'm not sure when mom started writing down things daily—how she felt, etc. Some days were lots better than others were. I think she was hoping all the pain would be gone once she got her new knees. It wasn't. She just had a different type of pain. She had a Memorial Day get together at her house. She was able to do more and more and got better as each week went by. By the time her 50th reunion rolled around in August she was doing really well.

Now, here it is, almost a year after the surgery. Only now, after a year, does she suggest to anyone facing knee replacement surgery that they have both knees done at once. It takes long time to feel confident that you made the right decision.

We all felt so helpless when we knew she was in pain or feeling down—none of us knew or could relate to how she was feeling. It would have been nice if she could have talked with someone who had the same surgery and they could have shared their experiences. I think that is what we hope to accomplish by writing this diary. Maybe in the future, someone else may be in mom's situation and can benefit or feel better once they've read this. At least it's a temporary way of feeling they're not alone.

Now when I ask if it hurts, mom says yes but in a different way than her arthritis. It is hard for her to explain. Some days I will call her and she is good, some days are bad. I think after nine months, she probably has more good days than bad. When she gets depressed about the pain, I remind her that before the surgery, she was basically homebound. The pain of walking prior to the surgery was so great that she often did not leave the house for days. Now, she may be in pain some days, but she can walk.

On New Years Day mom called me to say that this was the first day she can remember when her knees did not hurt at all! It looks like it will indeed take a full nine months to recover. And on January 2nd, she crossed her legs for the first time in years! Happy New Year. This was amazing to me and something I did not remembering her doing as long as I could remember!

Chapter Fourteen

Afterthoughts

There are a few after thoughts that come to mind. Be sure and do arm exercises and try not to rely on your arms as much. After all this time and going through problems with my arms after surgery—I do not use my arms to help me get off of a lower chair or couch. That is another thing. If you furniture is low—put a pillow or some kind of a "lifter" on the furniture—it is so much easier to get up from something higher—a straight chair is wonderful for me, but sometimes you really want some soft comfort.

One problem that has arisen is that I cannot kneel anymore. If I kneel the pain would be excruciating per the doctor. You cannot imagine how many things you do kneeling—that you now must find another way to do.

June of the following year—15 months after surgery. I went for a visit to the surgeons today—he indicated I was doing absolutely great. I asked him once again why I had such pain after surgery—did he cut nerves that created so much pain. One or two nerves were cut, but that was not the pain that I was feeling. He said the surgery was a major, major surgery and that alone caused the severe pain a person has. My x-rays looked excellent—and he told me that he wanted to see me once a year—but not really anything had to be done until approximately 12-15 years when another replacement might be possible. To this day I still exercise my legs, and of course, all the stairs I climb each day helps. I also have taken up walking. I have not accomplished a long distance in walking due to the fact that my hips hurt after a period of time—but, that is another story. I am very grateful to an accomplished surgeon, a great internist and all my family who helped me get through this lengthy process. How is that for a happy ending? I think it is a true happy ending.

About the Author

Ann Nohava was born and raised in Minnesota. She is the mother of six children. Ann is an active woman who did not want the pain of arthritic knees slowing her down. She hopes this book inspires anyone who reads it to take the plunge to a pain-free existence.

www.ingramcontent.com/pod-product-compliance
Lightning Source LLC
Chambersburg PA
CBHW030855180526
45163CB00004B/1588